Herbal Tinctures for Beginners: Natural Remedies for Healing Recipes and More

Kathy Wyatt

Published by CiJiRO Publishing, 2023.

While every precaution has been taken in the preparation of this book, the publisher assumes no responsibility for errors or omissions, or for damages resulting from the use of the information contained herein.

HERBAL TINCTURES FOR BEGINNERS: NATURAL REMEDIES FOR HEALING RECIPES AND MORE

First edition. July 5, 2023.

ISBN: 979-8223657545

Written by Kathy Wyatt.

Table of Contents

Chapter 1: Introduction to Herbal Tinctures 1

. Chapter 2: Benefits of Herbal Tinctures 4

Chapter 3: How to Make Herbal Tinctures 8

Chapter 4: Popular Herbs for Tincture Making 12

Chapter 5: Using Herbal Tinctures Effectively 20

Chapter 6: Herbal Tinctures for Common Health Concerns 23

Chapter 7: Exploring Versatile Herbal Tinctures 26

Chapter 8: Crafting Your Own Herbal Tinctures 29

Chapter 9: Exploring Advanced Herbal Tincture Techniques 32

Chapter 10: Storing and Preserving Your Herbal Tinctures 36

Chapter 11: Incorporating Herbal Tinctures into Your Daily Routine 39

Chapter 12: External Uses and Topical Applications of Herbal Tinctures.. 42

Chapter 13: Creative Applications of Herbal Tinctures for Holistic Well-Being 45

Chapter 14: Tincture Recipes 48

Immune-Boosting Tonic Tincture 49

Nervine Calm Tincture 50

Digestive Support Tincture 51

Respiratory Relief Tincture 52

Women's Balance Tincture 53

Stress Relief Tincture 54

Allergy Relief Tincture 55

Energy Boost Tincture 56

Joint Support Tincture 57

Digestive Calming Tincture 58

Immune Boosting Tonic 59

Anxiety Relief Tincture 60

Sleep Support Tincture 61

Hormonal Balance Tincture (for Women) 62

Focus and Clarity Tincture 63

Calming Nervous System Tincture 64

Respiratory Support Tincture 65

Mood Balancing Tincture 66

Hair and Scalp Nourishing Tincture 67

Circulation Support Tincture 68

Detox Support Tincture 69

Memory and Cognitive Function Tincture 70

Calming Sleep Tincture 71

Skin Healing Tincture 72

Joint Support Tincture 73

Eye Health Tincture 74

Digestive Bitters Tincture 75

Immune Boosting Tincture 76

Respiratory Support Tincture 77

Blood Sugar Balancing Tincture 78

Pancreatic Support Tincture 79

Ashwagandha and Lavender Stress Relief Tincture 80

Dong Quai and Mace Hormonal Balance Tincture (woman) 81

Peppermint Ginger Digestive Support Tincture 82

Energy Boost Tincture 2 83

Brain Health Tincture 2 84

Chapter 1: Introduction to Herbal Tinctures

In a world where modern medicine often takes center stage, it is easy to overlook the age-old wisdom of herbal remedies. But as we delve into the vast realm of natural healing, we discover a treasure trove of botanical wonders waiting to be explored. Among these treasures, herbal tinctures shine brightly as potent elixirs of health and vitality.

Herbal tinctures, also known as herbal extracts, are concentrated liquid preparations derived from various plants and herbs. They have been used for centuries across different cultures and civilizations, harnessing the power of nature to support wellness and treat a wide range of ailments. From soothing digestive discomfort to enhancing immune function, herbal tinctures offer a natural alternative for those seeking holistic approaches to health.

The process of creating herbal tinctures involves extracting the medicinal properties of plants by macerating them in a solvent, typically alcohol, although glycerin or vinegar can also be used. This method allows the plant's active constituents, such as alkaloids, flavonoids, and essential oils, to infuse into the liquid, resulting in a potent and concentrated herbal remedy.

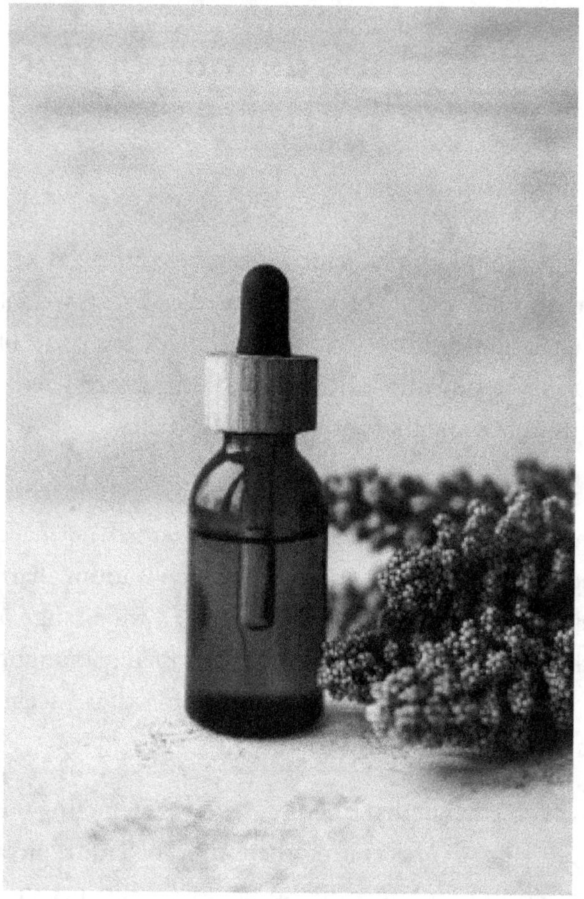

ONE OF THE ADVANTAGES of herbal tinctures is their ability to preserve the medicinal properties of plants for an extended period. Unlike dried herbs or teas that may lose potency over time, tinctures maintain their efficacy and potency for several years when stored properly. This longevity ensures that you always have a reliable herbal ally on hand whenever the need arises.

When it comes to choosing herbal tinctures, the options are as diverse as the plants themselves. Each herb possesses unique qualities and healing properties, and by combining different tinctures, we can create custom blends tailored to specific needs. Whether you're seeking relief from stress and anxiety, support for a healthy sleep routine, or a boost to your immune system, there's an herbal tincture waiting to assist you on your wellness journey.

It's important to note that while herbal tinctures offer a natural approach to healing, they are not without their considerations. As with any form of medicine, it is crucial to consult with a qualified healthcare professional before incorporating herbal tinctures into your wellness routine, especially if you have pre-existing health conditions or are taking prescription medications.

In the following chapters, we will explore a variety of herbal tinctures, their uses, and the science behind their therapeutic benefits. We will uncover the secrets of time-honored herbal traditions from around the world and shed light on the modern research that supports their efficacy. Together, we will embark on a captivating journey through the vibrant world of herbal medicine, where nature's wisdom intertwines with our quest for well-being.

So, dear reader, prepare to be captivated by the enchanting tales of botanical wonders and let the power of herbal tinctures awaken your senses. As we unlock the secrets of nature's medicine cabinet, we will discover the incredible potential that lies within the delicate petals, the resilient roots, and the aromatic leaves. Let us embark on this adventure together and may the world of herbal tinctures become a beacon of health and vitality in our lives.

. Chapter 2: Benefits of Herbal Tinctures

As we continue our exploration of the captivating world of herbal tinctures, we dive deeper into the realm of their remarkable benefits. These potent elixirs of nature possess an array of therapeutic properties that can support and enhance our overall well-being.

One of the key benefits of herbal tinctures is their capacity to deliver the potent and active components of plants in a concentrated form. The liquid nature of tinctures allows for efficient absorption by the body, ensuring that the beneficial compounds are readily available for utilization. This quick assimilation into our system enables us to experience the effects of herbal remedies more swiftly compared to other forms of herbal preparations.

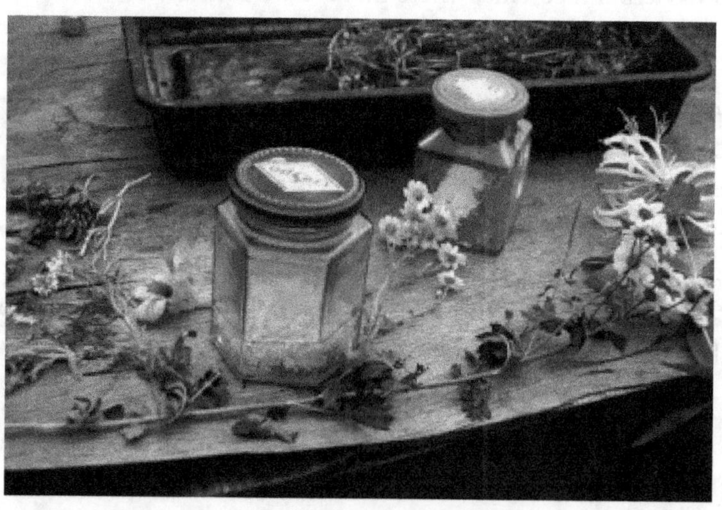

HERBAL TINCTURES OFFER a versatile approach to wellness, catering to a wide range of health concerns. Whether you are seeking relief from a specific condition or aiming to optimize your overall vitality, there is likely an herbal tincture suited to your needs. Let us explore some of the common benefits associated with these natural wonders.

- **Enhanced Immune Support:** Many herbal tinctures possess immune-boosting properties, helping to strengthen our body's defense mechanisms against external threats. From echinacea and elderberry to astragalus and medicinal mushrooms like reishi, these herbal allies can provide valuable support to our immune system, promoting resilience and overall well-being.
- **Digestive Harmony:** The digestive system plays a vital role in our overall health, and herbal tinctures can contribute to its optimal functioning. Herbs like peppermint, ginger, fennel, and chamomile have long been used to soothe digestive discomfort, alleviate indigestion, and promote a healthy digestive tract. Their calming and carminative properties can help ease bloating, gas, and other digestive disturbances.
- **Stress Relief and Emotional Well-being:** In the modern, fast-paced world we live in, stress and anxiety have become widespread challenges. Herbal tinctures offer a natural approach to finding balance and tranquility. Adaptogenic herbs such as ashwagandha, holy basil, and rhodiola rosea can help our bodies adapt to stress, promoting a sense of calm and emotional well-being. Additionally, herbs like passionflower and lemon balm possess relaxing properties that can support healthy sleep patterns.
- **Hormonal Balance:** Many individuals, particularly women, experience hormonal imbalances at different stages of life. Herbal tinctures can provide support in managing these

fluctuations. For example, chaste tree berry tincture has been traditionally used to support menstrual health and alleviate symptoms of premenstrual syndrome (PMS). Black cohosh tincture is known for its potential benefits during menopause, helping to alleviate hot flashes and hormonal discomfort.

- **Respiratory Health:** Herbal tinctures can offer relief and support for respiratory conditions. Eucalyptus, mullein, and marshmallow root are just a few examples of herbs known for their beneficial effects on the respiratory system. These tinctures can help soothe coughs, alleviate congestion, and support respiratory wellness.

It is essential to remember that while herbal tinctures can provide numerous benefits, they are not a one-size-fits-all solution. Each person's body is distinct, and what may be effective for one individual might not yield the same results for another. It is advisable to seek guidance from a knowledgeable healthcare professional or herbalist to identify the most appropriate herbal tinctures for your specific requirements.

In the forthcoming chapters, we will explore a variety of specific herbal tinctures in greater detail, delving into their historical uses, scientific research, and practical applications. We will unlock the secrets of their individual benefits, guiding you toward creating a personalized herbal tincture toolkit that aligns with your well-being goals.

So, come along with me for an enlightening journey through the remarkable benefits of herbal tinctures. Let the wisdom of nature's botanical allies enthrall you as we unlock their potential to support and enhance our physical, emotional, and spiritual health. May this chapter serve as a gateway to the myriad wonders that lie within the captivating realm of herbal medicine.

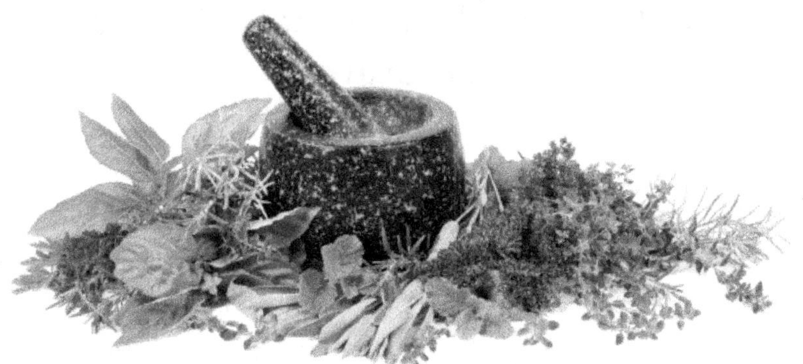

Chapter 3: How to Make Herbal Tinctures

Now that we have delved into the captivating benefits of herbal tinctures, it is time to uncover the art and science behind crafting these remarkable elixirs in the comfort of your own home. Making your own herbal tinctures allows you to harness the power of nature and tailor them to your specific needs. So, let us embark on a journey through the process of creating these botanical gems.

Before we dive into the step-by-step guide, it is important to gather the necessary materials and ingredients. Here's what you will need:

1. **Herbs:** Select the herbs that align with your desired outcomes. Ensure that they are of high quality and, if possible, organically grown or ethically sourced. You can choose to work with a single herb or create unique blends by combining different herbs.

2. **Alcohol:** Traditionally, herbal tinctures are made using alcohol as the solvent. Look for high-proof alcohol such as vodka, brandy, or rum, with at least 40% alcohol content (80 Proof) The alcohol acts as a preservative and helps extract the medicinal properties of the herbs. The preferred spirit to use in most cases is vodka. It is not necessary to buy a premium brand name, but don't get something that is an unknown brand as well. A middle of the road name brand would be fine. For the recipes in this book, we used vodka, but substituting a clear rum or unflavored brandy with the same 80 Proof (40% alcohol) would work fine as well.

3. **Glass Jar:** Choose a clean, sterilized glass jar with a tight-

fitting lid. Amber or dark-colored glass jars are preferred as they protect the tincture from light and help preserve its potency.

4. **Labels**: It is essential to label your tincture jars with the name of the herb, date of preparation, and any other relevant details. This ensures proper identification and allows you to keep track of your tincture collection.

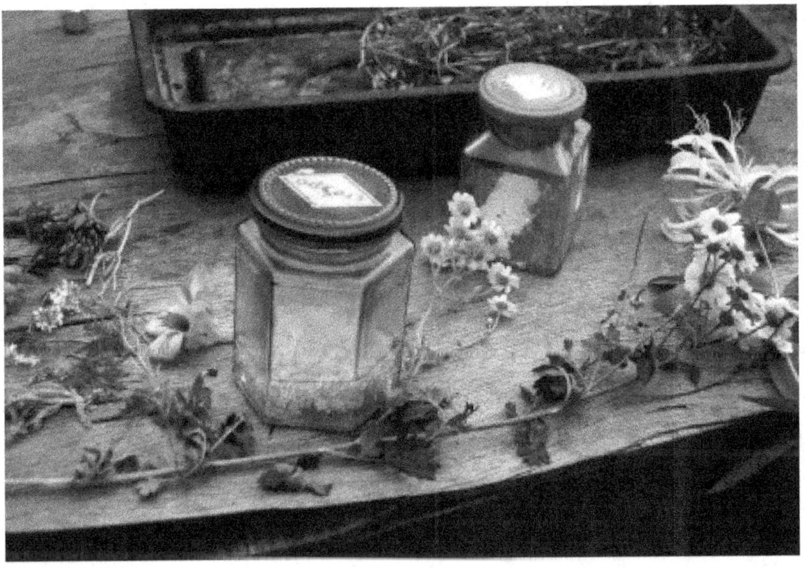

Now that you have assembled your materials, let's move on to the step-by-step process:

Step 1: Prepare the Herbs Begin by drying your fresh herbs if necessary. Remove any damaged or discolored parts and gently rinse the herbs to remove dirt or debris. Pat them dry and finely chop or grind them. If using dried herbs, crush or grind them to a coarse consistency. Remember, the quality of your tincture depends on the quality of your herbs, so handle them with care.

Step 2: Measure and Combine Measure the desired quantity of herbs and transfer them into the glass jar. It is recommended to start with a ratio of 1-part herbs to 4 or 5 parts alcohol for dried herbs, or 1-part herbs to 2 or 3 parts alcohol for fresh herbs. You can adjust the ratio based on the potency you desire.

Step 3: Pour the Alcohol Pour the alcohol over the herbs, ensuring that they are fully submerged. The alcohol should cover the herbs by at least an inch. Use a clean spoon or chopstick to gently stir the mixture, ensuring all the herbs are saturated.

Step 4: Seal and Store Secure the lid tightly on the jar. Store the jar away in a cool, dark pantry or cupboard from direct sunlight. This allows the tincture to macerate and extract the medicinal properties from the herbs. Shake the jar once or twice a day to encourage proper extraction.

Step 5: Steep and Strain Allow the tincture to steep for at least four to six weeks. The longer it steeps, the more potent the tincture will become. After the steeping period, strain the liquid through a fine mesh strainer or cheesecloth to remove the plant material. Squeeze the herbs to extract any remaining liquid.

Step 6: Bottle and Label Pour the strained tincture into dark-colored glass bottles for storage. Ensure the bottles are clean and sterilized. Label each bottle with the name of the herb, date of preparation, and any other relevant details. Proper labeling helps you stay organized and ensures you can easily identify your tinctures.

Congratulations! You have successfully created your own herbal tincture. Remember to store the bottles in a cool, dark place to maintain their potency.

It is crucial to note that the dosage of herbal tinctures varies depending on the herb and individual needs. To determine the suitable dosage for your specific needs, it is advisable to seek guidance from a knowledgeable healthcare professional or herbalist.

By making your own herbal tinctures, you embark on a journey of self-sufficiency and empower yourself to take control of your well-being. Experiment with different herbs, ratios, and blends to create personalized tinctures that cater to your unique health goals.

In the forthcoming chapters, we will explore specific herbs and their respective tincture-making processes in greater detail. So, dear reader, get ready to unlock the secrets of herbal alchemy as we delve into the world of individual herbs and their potent tinctures. May your tincture-making adventures be filled with joy, discovery, and the endless wonders of nature's healing treasures.

Chapter 4: Popular Herbs for Tincture Making

In our exploration of the captivating world of herbal tinctures, we turn our attention to some of the most popular herbs that are commonly used in tincture making. These botanical powerhouses have been cherished for their medicinal properties and have found their way into countless tincture formulations. Join us as we discover the wonders of these herbs and their potential to enhance our well-being.

- **Echinacea** (Echinacea purpurea): Echinacea is a beloved herb known for its immune-enhancing properties. Its tincture is commonly used to support the body's natural defenses, especially during times of seasonal challenges. Echinacea tincture is believed to stimulate the immune system and help shorten the duration of colds and flu.

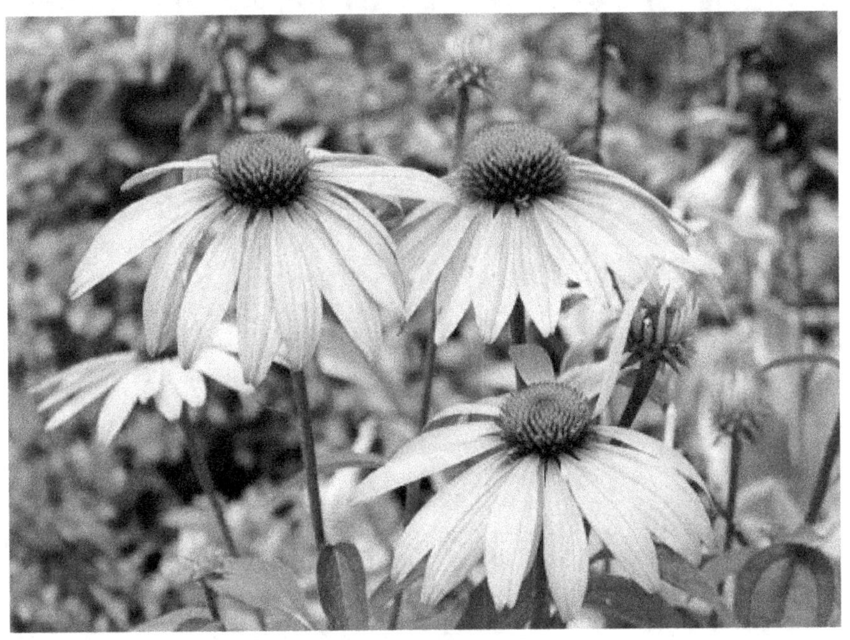

Echinacea

- **Chamomile** (Matricaria chamomilla): Chamomile tincture is celebrated for its calming and soothing effects. This herb has been used for centuries to promote relaxation, alleviate stress, and support healthy sleep patterns. Chamomile tincture can be a gentle remedy for those seeking tranquility in their daily lives.

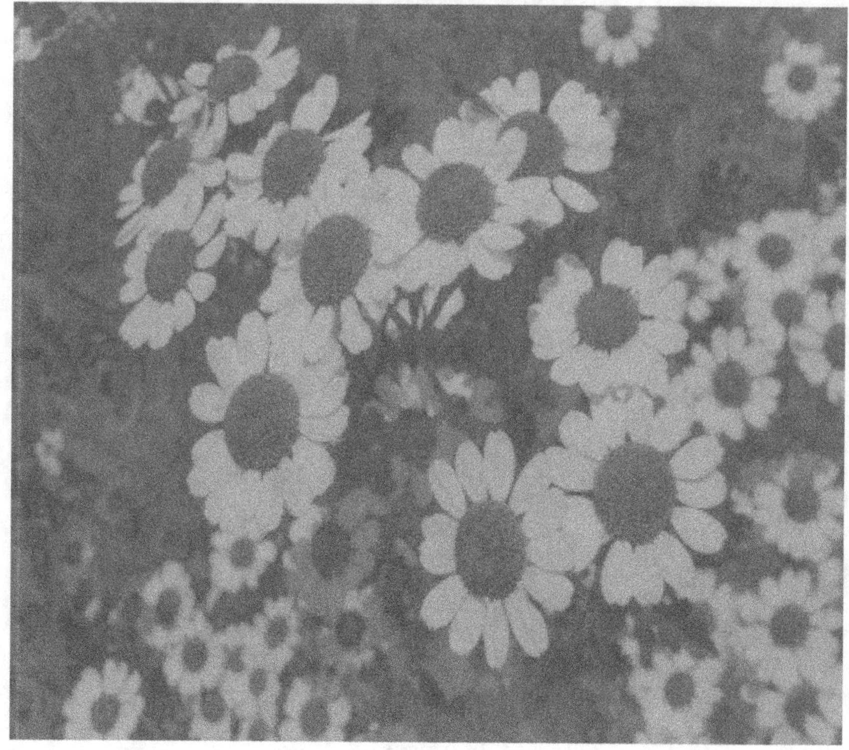

Chamomile

- Milk Thistle (Silybum marianum): Milk thistle is a powerful herb known for its liver-protective properties. The tincture derived from its seeds is often used to support liver health and detoxification. It is believed to have antioxidant and anti-inflammatory effects, making it a popular choice for those seeking to promote healthy function of the liver.

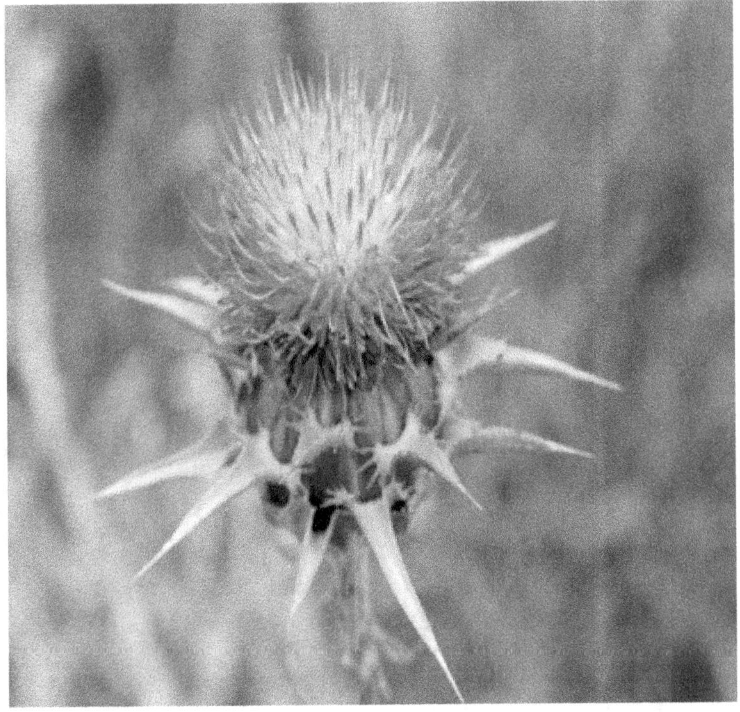

Milk Thistle

-
- St. John's Wort (Hypericum perforatum): St. John's Wort Tincture is revered for its potential benefits in supporting emotional well-being. This herb is commonly used to address symptoms of anxiety and mild to moderate depression. St. John's Wort has been found to increase the levels of serotonin; a neurotransmitter associated with mood regulation.

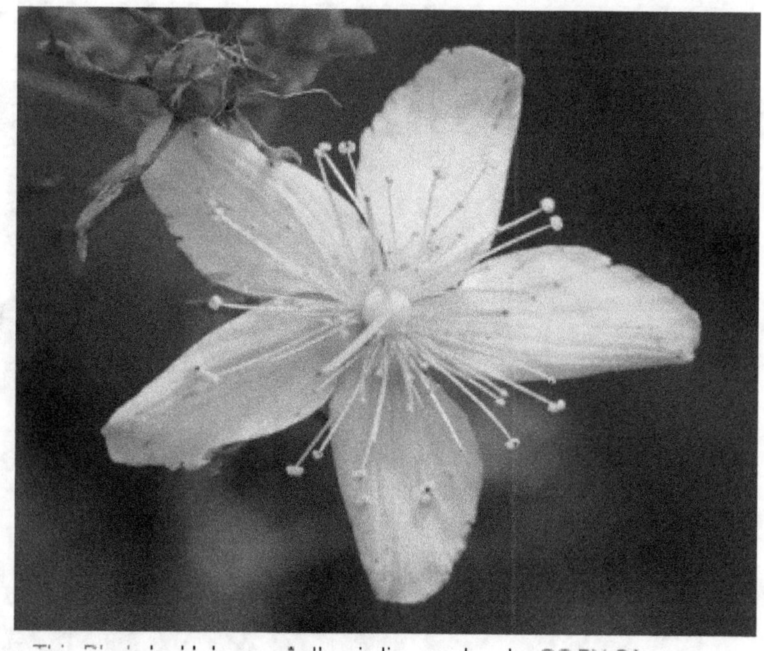

St. Johns Wort

- Valerian (Valeriana officinalis): Valerian tincture is a go-to herbal remedy for promoting relaxation and supporting a restful night's sleep. This herb has been used for centuries to ease nervous tension, anxiety, and sleep disturbances. Valerian tincture is known for its calming effects without causing grogginess the next day.

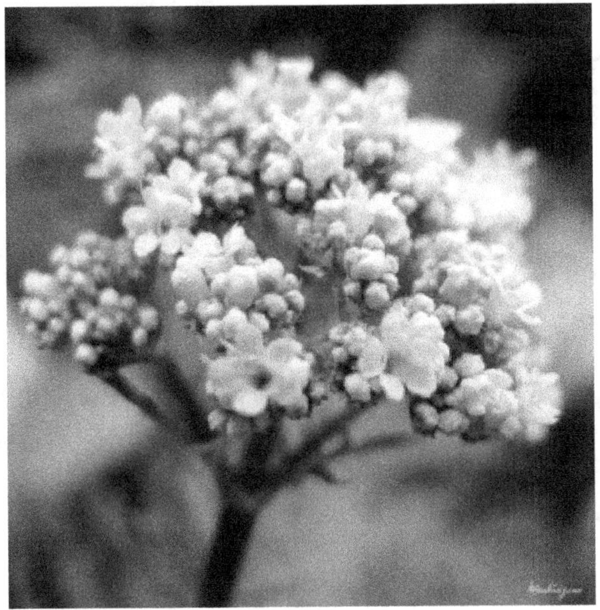

Valerian

- Ginger (Zingiber officinale): Ginger tincture is prized for its digestive benefits. This warming herb is often used to alleviate nausea, support healthy digestion, and ease gastrointestinal discomfort. Ginger tincture can be especially helpful for those experiencing motion sickness or digestive upset.
- Hawthorn (Crataegus spp.): Hawthorn tincture is valued for its cardiovascular benefits. This herb is known to support heart health, improve circulation, and promote overall cardiovascular well-being. Hawthorn tincture is believed to have antioxidant properties that help protect the heart from oxidative stress.

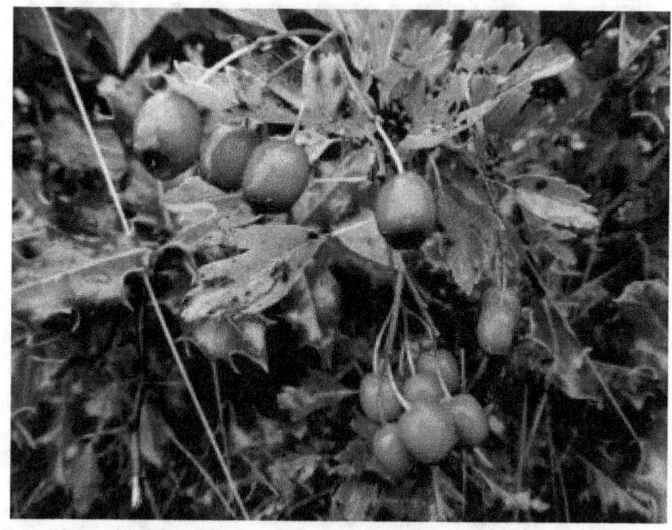

Hawthorn Berries

- Lavender (Lavandula spp.): Lavender tincture is cherished for its calming and balancing effects on the nervous system. This fragrant herb is often used to reduce stress, anxiety, and promote relaxation. Lavender tincture can be incorporated into self-care rituals, such as aromatic baths or massage oils.

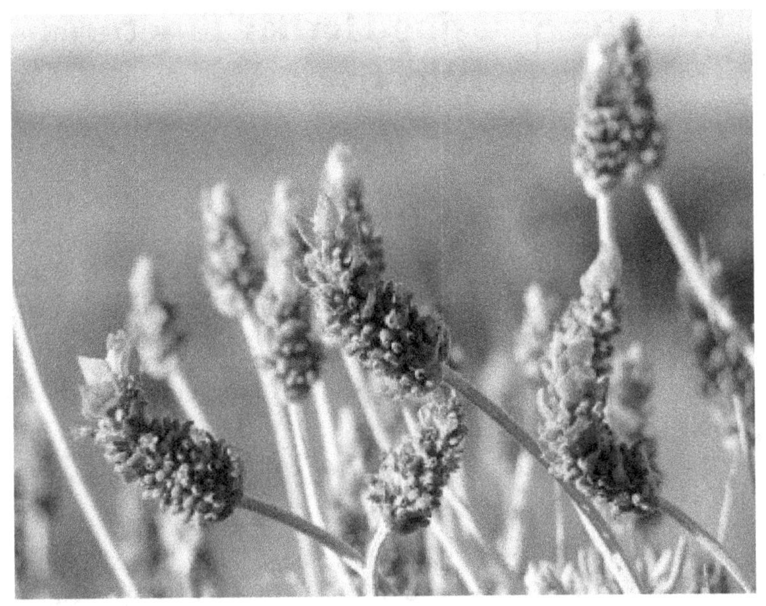

Lavender

THESE ARE JUST A FEW examples of the many herbs that can be transformed into potent tinctures. As you explore the world of herbal medicine, you will discover a vast array of plants and their unique properties. Remember to research each herb thoroughly, including potential contraindications and proper dosage recommendations, before creating your own tinctures.

In the next chapter, we will delve deeper into the fascinating world of specific herbal tinctures, their uses, and the scientific evidence supporting their effectiveness. Prepare to be amazed as we uncover the secrets of these natural remedies and their potential to revolutionize your well-being.

Chapter 5: Using Herbal Tinctures Effectively

Having explored the captivating world of herbal tinctures and the plethora of benefits they offer; it is essential to understand how to use these botanical elixirs effectively. Harnessing the power of herbal tinctures requires knowledge of proper dosage, administration methods, and considerations for optimal results. Join us as we delve into the art of using herbal tinctures effectively.

1. Dosage Guidelines: Determining the right dosage for herbal tinctures is crucial to ensure their safe and effective use. Dosages may vary depending on factors such as age, weight, health condition, and the specific herb being used. It is recommended to consult with a natural healthcare provider or herbalist to determine the best dosage for your individual needs.

2. Dilution: Herbal tinctures are typically concentrated extracts, and dilution is often necessary before consumption. Diluting the tincture in a small amount of water or juice can help minimize the strong taste and make it more palatable. Follow the dosage instructions provided by a knowledgeable source or refer to the recommendations on the tincture's label.

3. Sublingual Administration: Sublingual administration involves placing the tincture directly under the tongue for absorption through the sublingual glands. This method allows for rapid absorption of the herbal constituents into the bloodstream, bypassing the digestive system. Hold the tincture under your tongue for about 30 seconds to a minute before swallowing.

4. Custom Blending: One of the great advantages of herbal

tinctures is their versatility in creating custom blends. You can combine different tinctures to address specific health concerns or create a synergistic effect. However, exercise caution and seek guidance from a qualified herbalist to ensure compatibility and appropriate dosages when blending multiple tinctures.

5. Timing of Administration: The timing of tincture administration can impact their effectiveness. Some herbs are better taken on an empty stomach, while others are more suitable after meals. Pay attention to any specific instructions provided for the tincture you are using. If in doubt, consult a healthcare professional or refer to reputable herbal references for guidance.

6. Adherence to Recommended Duration: Follow the recommended duration of use for the specific herbal tincture you are using. Some tinctures are intended for short-term use, while others may be safely used long-term. Adhering to the recommended duration helps maintain the balance between the therapeutic benefits and potential risks associated with prolonged use.

7. Monitoring and Adjusting: As with any form of herbal medicine, it is important to monitor your body's response to the tincture. Observe for any adverse reactions or unexpected changes in symptoms. If necessary, adjust the dosage or discontinue use in consultation with a healthcare professional.

8. Integration with a Holistic Approach: Remember that herbal tinctures are just one facet of a holistic approach to well-being. They work best when combined with a healthy lifestyle, balanced diet, stress management techniques, regular exercise, and other supportive practices. Embrace a holistic mindset and integrate herbal tinctures into a comprehensive wellness plan.

By understanding and implementing these practices, you can effectively harness the power of herbal tinctures to support your health and well-being. Always prioritize safety, seek professional guidance, and be an active participant in your own health journey.

In the upcoming chapters, we will explore more specific applications of herbal tinctures, dive deeper into the science behind their efficacy, and shed light on additional strategies for incorporating these botanical wonders into your daily life. Prepare to unlock the full potential of herbal tinctures as we continue this enlightening journey together.

Chapter 6: Herbal Tinctures for Common Health Concerns

In this chapter, we will explore the fascinating realm of herbal tinctures and their application in addressing common health concerns. Herbal medicine has a rich history of providing natural remedies for various ailments, and tinctures offer a convenient and effective way to harness the healing properties of herbs. Join us as we uncover the potential of herbal tinctures for common health issues.

- Digestive Health: Herbal tinctures can be invaluable for promoting digestive well-being. Peppermint (Mentha x piperita) tincture, for instance, is known for its ability to ease symptoms of indigestion, bloating, and gas. Ginger (Zingiber officinale) tincture, with its warming properties, can help alleviate nausea and support healthy digestion. Chamomile (Matricaria chamomilla) tincture is beneficial for soothing digestive discomfort and promoting relaxation in the digestive system.
- Immune Support: When it comes to supporting the immune system, several herbal tinctures have gained recognition. Echinacea (Echinacea purpurea) tincture is known for its immune-enhancing properties, helping to strengthen the natural defenses of the body. Elderberry (Sambucus nigra) tincture has gained popularity for its potential to support immune health and reduce the severity of cold and flu symptoms. Astragalus (Astragalus membranaceus) tincture is traditionally used to enhance immune function and improve resistance to infections.
- Stress and Anxiety: Herbal tinctures can provide solace in

times of stress and anxiety. Valerian (Valeriana officinalis) tincture is renowned for its calming effects, helping to ease nervous tension and promote relaxation. Lemon balm (Melissa officinalis) tincture is another herb valued for its anxiolytic properties, promoting a sense of calm and balance. Passionflower (Passiflora incarnata) tincture has been used for centuries to alleviate anxiety and promote restful sleep.

- Sleep Support: Many individuals struggle with sleep issues, and herbal tinctures offer gentle remedies for promoting restful sleep. California poppy (Eschscholzia californica) tincture is known for its sedative properties, aiding in easing sleep disturbances, and promoting relaxation. Skullcap (Scutellaria lateriflora) tincture is another herb that can support a restful night's sleep, particularly for those experiencing nervous tension or racing thoughts before bed.

- Joint and Muscular Health: Herbal tinctures can be beneficial for promoting joint and muscular health. Turmeric (Curcuma longa) tincture, with its anti-inflammatory properties, is often used to alleviate joint pain and stiffness. Arnica (Arnica montana) tincture, when applied topically, can help relieve muscle soreness and inflammation. Devil's claw (Harpagophytum procumbens) tincture is traditionally used for its analgesic properties, supporting joint comfort and mobility.

- Respiratory Health: Certain herbal tinctures can provide support for respiratory health. Mullein (Verbascum thapsus) tincture is known for its soothing effects on the respiratory system and is often used to alleviate coughs and respiratory congestion. Thyme (Thymus vulgaris) tincture is valued for its antimicrobial properties and can be used to support respiratory health during seasonal challenges.

- Women's Health: Herbal tinctures offer support for various aspects of women's health. Vitex (Vitex agnus-castus) tincture is commonly used to promote hormonal balance and alleviate symptoms of premenstrual syndrome (PMS). Black cohosh (Actaea racemosa) tincture has been traditionally used to ease menopausal symptoms such as hot flashes and mood swings. Raspberry leaf (Rubus idaeus) tincture is known for its toning effect on the uterus and can be beneficial during pregnancy and childbirth.

These are just a few examples of the vast array of herbal tinctures available to address common health concerns. Remember, it is essential to consult with a qualified doctor or herbalist to determine the most suitable tinctures and dosages for your specific needs. Embrace the power of nature as you explore the world of herbal tinctures and discover their remarkable potential to support your well-being.

In the upcoming chapters, we will further explore specific herbs and their tincture formulations for targeted health concerns, allowing you to unlock the full potential of herbal medicine. Prepare to embark on a journey of healing and transformation as we delve deeper into the world of herbal tinctures for holistic wellness.

Chapter 7: Exploring Versatile Herbal Tinctures

In this chapter, we embark on an exploration of versatile herbal tinctures that offer a wide range of applications and benefits. These remarkable botanical extracts possess diverse properties that can be utilized for various health concerns and wellness goals. Join us as we uncover the versatility and potential of these herbal tinctures.

- Holy Basil (Ocimum sanctum) Tincture: Also known as Tulsi, Holy Basil is an esteemed herb in Ayurvedic medicine. Holy Basil tincture offers adaptogenic properties, helping the body adapt to stress and promote overall balance. It is valued for its potential to support mental clarity, enhance immune function, and promote respiratory health. Holy Basil tincture can be incorporated into daily wellness routines to foster resilience and vitality.
- Lemon Verbena (Aloysia citrodora) Tincture: Lemon Verbena is a citrus-scented herb known for its refreshing and uplifting qualities. Lemon Verbena tincture offers a delightful burst of flavor and aroma. It is often used to support digestive health, ease indigestion, and promote healthy liver function. Additionally, Lemon Verbena tincture can be enjoyed as a calming and aromatic addition to herbal tea blends.
- Nettle (Urtica dioica) Tincture: Nettle is a versatile herb with a long history of traditional use. Nettle tincture is renowned for its potential benefits in supporting allergy relief, promoting healthy inflammatory response, and nourishing the body with essential vitamins and minerals. It can be used as a daily tonic to support overall well-being and vitality.

- Hawthorn (Crataegus spp.) Tincture: Hawthorn, a beloved herb for cardiovascular health, offers versatile benefits in tincture form. Hawthorn tincture is traditionally used to support heart health, enhance circulation, and promote healthy blood pressure levels. It is cherished for its potential to strengthen the cardiovascular system and support overall cardiovascular well-being.

- Calendula (Calendula officinalis) Tincture: Calendula, with its vibrant and cheerful flowers, has been treasured for centuries for its soothing and healing properties. Calendula tincture is often used topically to support skin health, soothe minor irritations, and promote wound healing. It can be added to natural skincare preparations or used as a gentle herbal remedy for skin concerns.

- Ashwagandha (Withania somnifera) Tincture: Ashwagandha, an ancient herb in Ayurvedic medicine, is renowned for its adaptogenic qualities. Ashwagandha tincture is prized for its potential to support stress management, promote mental well-being, and enhance energy levels. It can be a valuable ally in navigating the challenges of modern life, helping to restore balance and vitality.

- Dandelion (Taraxacum officinale) Tincture: Dandelion, often considered a humble weed, possesses remarkable properties for liver support and detoxification. Dandelion tincture is utilized to promote healthy liver function, aid in digestion, and support overall detoxification processes in the body. It can be incorporated into cleansing protocols or used as a gentle tonic for overall liver health.

- Passionflower (Passiflora incarnata) Tincture: Passionflower, with its intricate and beautiful blossoms, offers calming and soothing properties. Passionflower tincture is known for its potential to alleviate anxiety, reduce nervous tension, and support restful sleep. It can be a valuable addition to relaxation rituals, promoting a sense of tranquility and inner peace.

These are just a few examples of versatile herbal tinctures available to support various aspects of health and well-being. As you explore the world of herbal tinctures, remember to source high-quality products, and consult with a qualified healthcare professional or herbalist for personalized guidance.

In the following chapters, we will delve into the applications and benefits of specific herbal tinctures, allowing you to harness their versatility and unlock their full potential for your journey toward optimal health and vitality. Get ready to expand your herbal repertoire and embrace the magic of these botanical wonders.

Chapter 8: Crafting Your Own Herbal Tinctures

In this chapter, we venture into the world of herbal alchemy and discover the art of crafting your own herbal tinctures. Creating your own tinctures allows you to have full control over the quality, ingredients, and potency of these botanical extracts. Join us as we dive into the process of crafting herbal tinctures and unlock the joy of homemade remedies.

- **Gathering and Preparing Herbs:** Begin by selecting high-quality herbs for your tincture. Whether you choose fresh herbs from your garden or dried herbs from reputable sources, ensure they are free from pesticides or contaminants. If using fresh herbs, gently wash and pat them dry. If using dried herbs, crush or chop them to increase surface area and enhance extraction.

- **Choosing the Solvent:** The solvent, usually alcohol or a mixture of alcohol and water, is responsible for extracting the beneficial compounds from the herbs. High-proof alcohol such as vodka, brandy, or grain alcohol (at least 40-50% alcohol content) is commonly used for tincture making. The alcohol acts as a preservative and facilitates the extraction of active constituents. If desired, you can adjust the alcohol-to-water ratio based on the herb and desired strength.

- **Jar Selection:** Put your tincture in a glass jar with a snug-fitting lid. Clear glass or amber glass jars are commonly used, as they provide visibility and protection from light. Ensure the jar is clean and sterilized before use to maintain the integrity of the tincture.

- **Herb-to-Solvent Ratio:** The herb-to-solvent ratio determines the potency of your tincture. As a general guideline, a 1:5 ratio is often used, meaning one part herb to five parts solvent by volume. However, you can adjust the ratio based on the herb's strength and your desired potency. Experimentation and personal preference play a role in finding the right balance.

- **Maceration Process:** Place the prepared herbs in the glass jar and cover them with the chosen solvent. Ensure the herbs are fully submerged, leaving some headspace to allow for expansion during maceration. Seal the jar tightly and give it a gentle shake to distribute the solvent evenly. Store the jar in a cool pantry or cupboard away from the sun and let the mixture macerate for about 4 to 6 weeks. During this time, the alcohol will extract the medicinal compounds from the herbs.

- **Regular Agitation:** While the tincture is macerating, it's beneficial to agitate the jar every few days. This helps facilitate the extraction process and ensures thorough mixing of the herb and solvent. Give the jar a gentle shake or stir to promote optimal extraction.

- **Straining and Pressing:** After the maceration period, it's time to strain and press the tincture. Use a fine-mesh strainer or cheesecloth to separate the liquid from the herb solids. Squeeze or press the herb residue to extract any remaining tincture. Collect the strained liquid in a clean glass container, preferably amber glass bottles, and label them with the herb name and date of preparation.

- **Storage and Aging:** Store your homemade tinctures in a cool, dark place to preserve their potency. Amber glass bottles offer protection from light, which can degrade the tincture over time. Properly stored tinctures can last for several years, retaining their efficacy.

- **Dosage and Usage:** Consult reputable herbal references or a qualified herbalist to determine the appropriate dosage for your specific tincture. Dosage may vary depending on the herb's strength and intended use. Start with a low dosage and gradually increase if needed. Tinctures can be taken directly by mouth or diluted in water or juice.

Crafting your own herbal tinctures is a rewarding and empowering journey. It allows you to develop a deeper connection with the plants and customize remedies to suit your unique needs. Embrace the art of herbal alchemy and let your creativity flourish as you experiment with different herbs and formulations. The possibilities are endless, and the joy of crafting your own herbal tinctures awaits you.

Chapter 9: Exploring Advanced Herbal Tincture Techniques

In this chapter, we delve into the realm of advanced herbal tincture techniques, taking our tincture-making skills to the next level. These techniques offer innovative approaches to extract and enhance the potency of herbal constituents. Join us as we explore the fascinating world of advanced herbal tincture techniques and expand our knowledge of botanical alchemy.

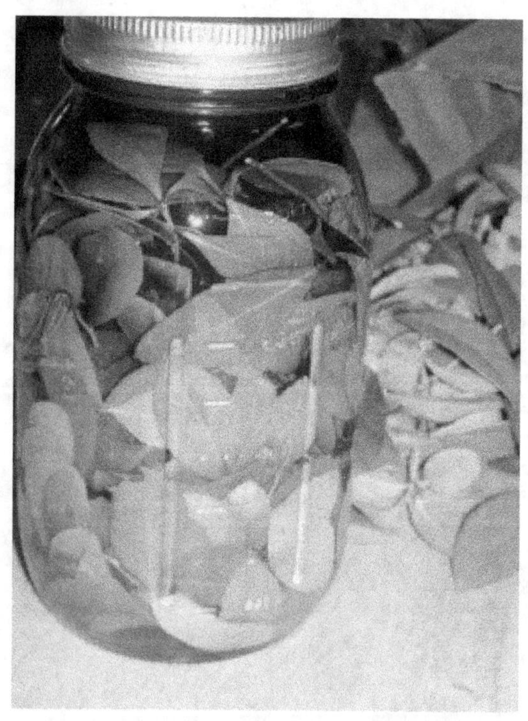

- Double Extraction Method: The double extraction method is employed when working with herbs that contain both water-soluble and alcohol-soluble compounds. This technique combines the benefits of both water and alcohol extraction to yield a comprehensive tincture. Start by macerating the herbs in alcohol as usual. After the alcohol extraction period, strain the liquid and set it aside. Then, take the spent herb material and prepare a decoction by simmering it in water. Afterward, strain the decoction and combine it with the alcohol extract. The resulting tincture will contain a broader spectrum of medicinal constituents.

- Spagyric Tinctures: Spagyric tinctures are a fascinating aspect of alchemical herbalism. This technique involves a three-step process: separation, purification, and recombination. First, the plant material is burned to create a white ash known as the "salts." The remaining ash is dissolved in water, filtered, and purified. Meanwhile, the liquid extraction (often alcohol) of the plant material is also prepared. Finally, the purified salts and the liquid extract are combined, creating a spagyric tincture that incorporates the mineral salts back into the tincture. This technique aims to capture the complete essence of the plant, including its mineral components.

- Vibrational or Energetic Infusion: Vibrational or energetic infusion techniques involve imbuing the tincture with specific energetic qualities. This can be achieved by incorporating various methods such as sound, intention, or gemstone infusion. Sound infusion involves exposing the tincture to specific frequencies or vibrations, such as chanting or using singing bowls. Intention infusion involves consciously directing positive intentions or affirmations into the tincture during preparation. Gemstone infusion involves placing gemstones or crystals in the tincture to infuse it with their energetic properties. These techniques aim to enhance the vibrational qualities of the tincture for a more holistic approach to healing.

- Lunar or Solar Infusion: Lunar and solar infusions harness the energetic influences of the moon and sun, respectively, during the tincture-making process. Lunar infusion involves placing the tincture mixture under moonlight for a designated period, typically aligning with the phases of the moon. This method is believed to imbue the tincture with the subtle energies associated with the lunar cycle. Solar infusion, on the other hand, involves exposing the tincture to sunlight, harnessing the vibrant energy of the sun. These techniques add an additional dimension to tincture preparation, connecting with the natural rhythms of the celestial bodies.

- Sequential Extraction: Sequential extraction is a technique used to create tinctures that capture the sequential release of medicinal constituents from the plant material. It involves macerating the herb in a series of solvents with increasing polarity. This allows for the extraction of different groups of compounds, such as essential oils, water-soluble constituents, and alcohol-soluble constituents. Each solvent extraction is performed separately, and the resulting extracts are combined to create a comprehensive tincture with a wider spectrum of active compounds.

- Fermentation: Fermentation is a transformative process that can be applied to herbal tincture making. This technique involves allowing the tincture mixture to undergo controlled fermentation, facilitated by the introduction of beneficial microorganisms. The fermentation process can enhance the extraction of certain compounds, promote the breakdown of complex constituents, and create new bioactive compounds. Fermented tinctures often develop unique flavors and aromas, along with potential probiotic benefits.

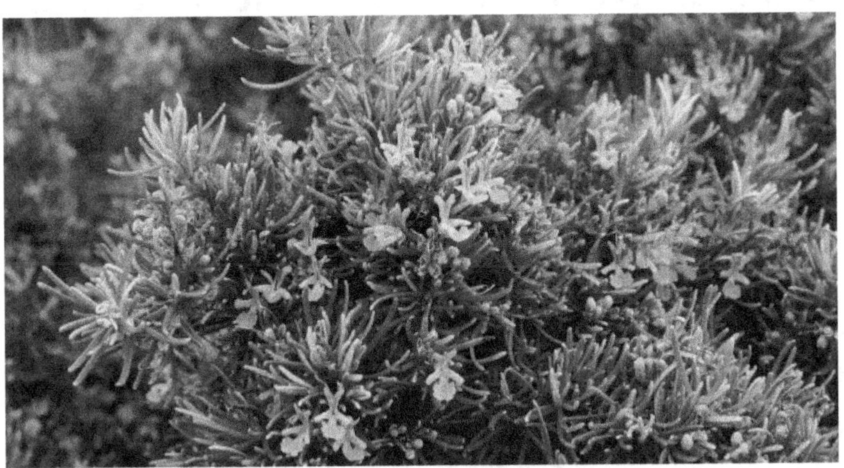

BY EXPLORING THESE advanced herbal tincture techniques, you can expand your understanding and appreciation for the art of tincture making. These methods provide opportunities to create unique and potent remedies while tapping into the deeper aspects of herbal alchemy. Experiment with these techniques and let your creativity flow as you unlock new dimensions in your herbal journey.

Chapter 10: Storing and Preserving Your Herbal Tinctures

In this chapter, we explore the essential practices for storing and preserving your precious herbal tinctures. Proper storage ensures the longevity and potency of your tinctures, allowing you to enjoy their benefits for an extended period. Join us as we delve into the world of tincture storage and preservation techniques.

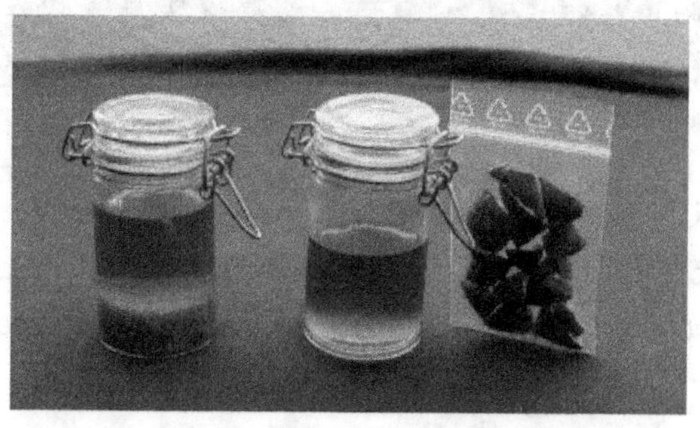

- Choose the Right Containers: Selecting the appropriate containers for storing your herbal tinctures is crucial. Amber glass bottles are highly recommended as they provide protection from light, which can degrade the potency of the tincture over time. Ensure the bottles have airtight lids or dropper caps to prevent air exposure and leakage. Consider using different-sized bottles to accommodate varying tincture quantities.

- Labeling and Dating: Properly labeling your herbal tinctures is essential for easy identification and monitoring their shelf life. Clearly write the name of the herb, the date of preparation, and any additional relevant information such as the alcohol percentage or dosage recommendations. This helps you keep track of the tinctures and use them in a timely manner.

- Storage Conditions: To maintain the potency and quality of your herbal tinctures, store them in optimal conditions. Choose a cool, dark, and dry location away from direct sunlight, heat sources, and humidity. Fluctuations in temperature and exposure to light can degrade the tincture over time. A pantry, cupboard, or drawer can be ideal storage spots for your tinctures.

- Avoid Contamination: To prevent contamination, it is crucial to handle tinctures with clean hands and use clean utensils when dispensing them. Avoid touching the dropper or bottle opening with your fingers to minimize the introduction of bacteria. Additionally, ensure that the containers are thoroughly cleaned and sterilized before transferring tinctures into them.

- Minimize Air Exposure: Air exposure can lead to oxidation and the loss of volatile compounds in the tincture. When using a dropper, make sure to expel any excess air from the dropper before sealing the bottle. This reduces the amount of air in the bottle, minimizing oxidation. Always tighten the lid or cap securely after each use to limit air exposure.

- Tincture Shelf Life: Herbal tinctures, when stored properly, can maintain their potency for an extended period. However, it is important to note that the shelf life can vary depending on the herb and the extraction method used. As a general guideline, alcohol-based tinctures can last for several years, while glycerin-based tinctures have a shorter shelf life. It is recommended to consume or replace tinctures within 1 to 3 years to ensure optimal freshness and efficacy.

- Checking for Spoilage: Regularly inspect your tinctures for any signs of spoilage or degradation. Look for changes in color, texture, or smell. If you notice any mold growth, cloudiness, or unpleasant odor, discard the tincture immediately, as it may indicate contamination or deterioration. Trust your senses and prioritize safety when using herbal tinctures.

By following these storage and preservation practices, you can ensure the longevity and effectiveness of your herbal tinctures. Properly stored tinctures offer reliable remedies for your health and wellness needs. Embrace the art of tincture storage and care and enjoy the benefits of your homemade botanical extracts for years to come.

Chapter 11: Incorporating Herbal Tinctures into Your Daily Routine

In this chapter, we explore the many ways you can incorporate herbal tinctures into your daily routine to maximize their benefits and make them a seamless part of your wellness journey. Herbal tinctures offer a convenient and effective way to harness the healing power of plants. Join us as we discover practical tips and creative ideas for integrating herbal tinctures into your everyday life.

- Start with a Clear Intention: Before incorporating herbal tinctures into your routine, it's helpful to set a clear intention for their use. Reflect on your health goals, whether it's boosting immunity, promoting relaxation, or addressing specific concerns. Having a focused intention can guide you in selecting the appropriate tinctures and determining the dosage and frequency of use.
- Create a Daily Ritual: Establishing a daily ritual around taking your herbal tinctures can enhance the experience and make it more meaningful. Find a quiet and comfortable space where you can take a few moments to connect with yourself. Take a deep breath, express gratitude for the healing power of nature, and set your intentions for the day. Incorporate your tincture into this ritual, allowing it to become a mindful act of self-care.
- Timing and Consistency: Consistency is key when incorporating herbal tinctures into your routine. Determine the best times to take your tinctures based on their specific properties and your personal preferences. Some tinctures are best taken in the morning to invigorate and energize, while others may be more suitable for evening use to promote

relaxation and sleep. Set reminders or incorporate them into existing daily rituals to ensure regular intake.

- Dilute in Water or Tea: If the taste or potency of a tincture is too strong for you, consider diluting it in a small amount of water or herbal tea. This can make the experience more palatable while still allowing the tincture to be effective. Experiment with different combinations to find the right balance of flavor and efficacy.

- Mix with Other Beverages or Foods: Incorporating herbal tinctures into other beverages or foods is another creative way to enjoy their benefits. Add some drops of your tincture to your favorite smoothie, juice, or herbal elixir. You can also drizzle tinctures over salads, stir them into yogurt or oatmeal, or infuse them into salad dressings or sauces. Get creative and explore different culinary possibilities.

- Customize Your Tincture Blend: Another exciting aspect of herbal tinctures is the ability to create personalized blends that target specific health concerns or support your overall well-being. Experiment with combining different tinctures to create your unique formulations. Consult reputable herbal references or work with a qualified herbalist to ensure proper dosage and compatibility.

- Keep a Tincture Journal: Maintaining a tincture journal can be a valuable practice in tracking your experiences and noting the effects of different tinctures. Record the tinctures you take, their dosages, and any observations or changes you notice in your physical, emotional, or mental well-being. This helps you gain insights into which tinctures work best for you and allows for adjustments as needed.

- Share the Knowledge: If you find value in incorporating herbal tinctures into your daily routine, consider sharing your knowledge and experiences with others. Discuss the benefits of tinctures with friends, family, or community members who may be interested in natural remedies. Encourage them to explore the world of herbal tinctures and offer guidance based on your own experiences.

By incorporating herbal tinctures into your daily routine, you embrace the power of plants and nourish your well-being. Let these potent botanical extracts become an integral part of your self-care practices, supporting you on your journey toward optimal health and vitality.

Chapter 12: External Uses and Topical Applications of Herbal Tinctures

In this chapter, we explore the diverse ways in which herbal tinctures can be used externally for topical applications. While herbal tinctures are commonly taken internally, their therapeutic properties can also be harnessed for external use. Join us as we delve into the realm of external applications and discover the versatility of herbal tinctures in promoting skin health, soothing discomfort, and supporting overall well-being.

- Herbal-Infused Oils: One of the most popular ways to utilize herbal tinctures externally is by creating herbal-infused oils. This involves combining the tincture with a carrier oil, like jojoba or olive oil, to properly extract and preserve the medicinal properties of the herbs. To make an herbal-infused oil, simply mix a measured amount of herbal tincture with the carrier oil, ensuring that the tincture is well incorporated. The resulting infused oil can be used for massage, skincare, hair care, and more.
- Skin Care Applications: Herbal tinctures can be valuable additions to your skincare routine. Dilute a few drops of tincture in water or aloe vera gel to create a soothing and refreshing facial toner. Apply the mixture to your skin using a cotton pad or spritz it onto your face. Some herbs, such as calendula and chamomile, are renowned for their calming and rejuvenating properties, making them ideal choices for skincare applications.
- Compresses and Poultices: Herbal tinctures can be incorporated into compresses and poultices to address specific skin conditions or discomfort. To create a compress, dilute the

tincture in warm water and soak a clean cloth or towel in the mixture. Apply the compress to the affected area for a soothing and therapeutic effect. Poultices involve creating a paste-like mixture by combining powdered herbs, herbal tinctures, and a binding agent, such as clay or flaxseed meal. Apply the poultice directly to the skin, cover with a cloth, and leave it on for the recommended time.

- Muscle and Joint Support: Herbal tinctures can be beneficial in promoting muscle and joint health. Create a massage oil by mixing a few drops of tincture with a carrier oil, such as coconut oil or almond oil. Gently massage the oil into the affected area to alleviate discomfort and support relaxation. Popular herbs for muscle and joint support include arnica, St. John's wort, and cayenne.

- Scalp and Hair Care: Herbal tinctures can also be used to promote scalp and hair health. Combine a few drops of tincture with a carrier oil, such as castor oil or argan oil, and massage the mixture into your scalp. This can help nourish the scalp, promote hair growth, and address common scalp conditions. Additionally, you can add some drops of tincture to your regular shampoo or conditioner for an added herbal boost.

- Mouth Rinse and Gargle: Certain herbal tinctures possess antimicrobial and soothing properties that make them suitable for oral care. Dilute a few drops of tincture in warm water and use the mixture as a mouth rinse or gargle. This can help freshen breath, soothe oral discomfort, and promote oral hygiene. Herbs like peppermint, sage, and myrrh are commonly used in oral care tinctures.

- Aromatherapy Applications: Some herbal tinctures have aromatic qualities that make them perfect for aromatherapy applications. Add a few drops of tincture to a diffuser or mix them with a carrier oil for use in massage or bath blends. Inhaling the aromatic compounds can promote relaxation, uplift the mood, and enhance overall well-being.

- Safety Considerations: While external use of herbal tinctures is generally safe, it's important to exercise caution and conduct a patch test before applying tinctures to larger areas of the skin. It is important to note that each person's body reacts differently to various herbs. Therefore, it is possible for individuals to have sensitivities or allergies to certain herbs. If you happen to experience any adverse reactions while using herbal tinctures, it is crucial to discontinue their use immediately. In such cases, it is highly recommended to consult a qualified healthcare professional who can provide appropriate guidance and support. Remember, your well-being is of utmost importance, and seeking professional advice ensures your safety and health.
- By exploring the external uses and topical applications of herbal tinctures, you open a world of possibilities for harnessing their therapeutic properties. Experiment with different herbs, formulations, and methods to find what works best for you. Embrace the holistic benefits of herbal tinctures and let them enhance your external well-being.

Chapter 13: Creative Applications of Herbal Tinctures for Holistic Well-Being

In this chapter, we embark on a journey of exploration into the creative applications of herbal tinctures for holistic well-being. While herbal tinctures are commonly known for their internal and external uses, there are numerous other ways to incorporate them into your daily life. Join us as we discover innovative and imaginative ways to utilize herbal tinctures for a well-rounded approach to health and wellness.

- Herbal Bath Soaks: Transform your bathing experience into a soothing and aromatic ritual by adding herbal tinctures to your bathwater. Mix a few droppers full of tincture with Epsom salts or sea salts and sprinkle the blend into your warm bath. Immerse yourself in the fragrant waters and allow the therapeutic properties of the herbs to envelop your senses. This is an excellent way to promote relaxation, ease muscle tension, and enhance overall well-being.
- Herbal Inhalations: Harness the power of herbal tinctures through inhalation to support respiratory health and invigorate the senses. Add a few drops of tincture to a bowl of hot water and cover your head with a towel to create a steam tent. Breathe deeply, allowing the herbal steam to penetrate your respiratory system. Eucalyptus, peppermint, and lavender are popular choices for inhalations due to their refreshing and clarifying properties.
- Herbal Infused Honey: Combine the sweetness of honey with the medicinal properties of herbal tinctures by creating your own herbal-infused honey. Mix a measured amount of tincture with raw, unprocessed honey and stir until well blended. Use

this infused honey to sweeten beverages, drizzle over yogurt or oatmeal, or enjoy it by the spoonful. The honey acts as a natural preservative, preserving the potency of the herbs while adding a delightful flavor.

- Herbal Room Sprays: Elevate the ambiance of your living space and enjoy the benefits of herbal tinctures by creating homemade room sprays. Dilute a few droppers full of tincture in water and pour the mixture into a spray bottle. Mist the herbal spray throughout your home, office, or any space you wish to freshen. This allows the aromatic properties of the herbs to purify the air and create a pleasant environment.

- Herbal Infused Vinegars: Add a tangy and herbal twist to your culinary creations by infusing vinegars with herbal tinctures. Combine a measured amount of tincture with apple cider vinegar or white wine vinegar and let the mixture steep for several weeks in a cool, dark place. The resulting infused vinegar can be used in dressings, marinades, and sauces, imparting the flavors and benefits of the herbs into your culinary delights.

- Herbal Energy Boosters: Give your energy levels a natural lift by incorporating herbal tinctures into energy-boosting concoctions. Mix a dropper full of tincture with your favorite herbal tea or blend it into a homemade energy drink. Herbs like ginseng, eleuthero, and schisandra are known for their revitalizing properties, providing a sustainable source of energy throughout the day.

- Herbal Meditation and Rituals: Enhance your meditation and ritual practices by incorporating the vibrational energy of herbal tinctures. Before starting your meditation or ritual, anoint yourself with a few drops of tincture on your wrists, temples, or heart center. The aroma and energetic qualities of the herbs can help deepen your connection with the present moment, promote clarity, and facilitate spiritual experiences.

- Herbal Sleep Support: Create a soothing bedtime routine by utilizing herbal tinctures to promote restful sleep. Mix a dropper full of tincture with warm milk, herbal tea, or a calming elixir before bed. Herbs like chamomile, passionflower, and valerian are renowned for their relaxing properties, helping you unwind and prepare for a restorative night's sleep.

- Herbal Potpourri and Sachets: Fill your living spaces with the delightful scents of dried herbs infused with tinctures by creating herbal potpourri or sachets. Combine dried herbs, flowers, and spices with a few drops of tincture in a bowl and let them sit for a few days to absorb the herbal essence. Place the mixture in small sachets or bowls around your home to enjoy the natural fragrance and reap the benefits of aromatherapy.

- Herbal Gemstone Elixirs: Combine the energetic properties of gemstones with the healing qualities of herbal tinctures by creating herbal gemstone elixirs. Place a cleansed gemstone, such as amethyst, rose quartz, or clear quartz, in a glass container with a measured amount of tincture. Fill the container with purified water and let it sit in sunlight or moonlight for a few hours. The resulting elixir can be taken orally or used topically, allowing you to experience the synergistic effects of the gemstone and herbal energies.

Incorporating herbal tinctures into creative applications expands the possibilities for holistic well-being. Embrace your imagination, experiment with different herbs, and let your creativity guide you as you explore the multifaceted uses of herbal tinctures. Discover new ways to enhance your daily life and cultivate a deeper connection with the healing power of nature.

Chapter 14: Tincture Recipes

These tinctures are not meant to prevent, cure, or treat any disease. Always check with your doctor or healthcare professional before taking these tinctures, as there may be potential for drug interactions.

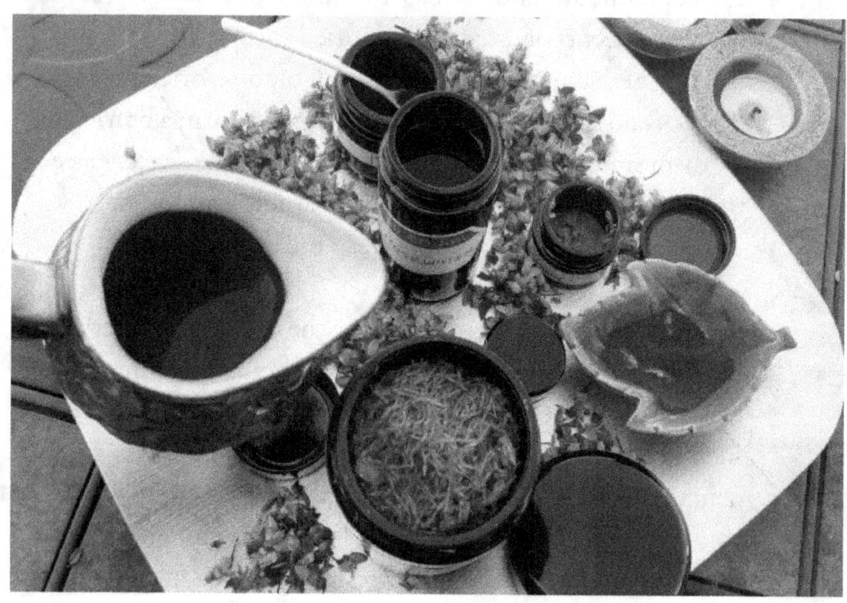

Immune-Boosting Tonic Tincture

Description: This immune-boosting tincture combines echinacea, elderberries, astragalus, and rose hips to provide a potent tonic for strengthening the immune system.

Ingredients:

- 2 tablespoons dried echinacea root
- 1 tablespoon dried astragalus root
- 1 tablespoon dried elderberries
- 1 tablespoon dried rose hips
- 1 cup vodka

Method:

1. Combine all the dried herbs in a glass jar.
2. Pour vodka over the herbs, ensuring they are fully covered.
3. Seal the jar tightly and shake well.
4. Store in a cool, dark cupboard for 4-6 weeks, shaking once daily.
5. Strain into a clean bottle.
6. Take 1-2 teaspoons daily to support immune health.

Nervine Calm Tincture

Description: This nervine calm tincture combines lemon balm, chamomile, passionflower, and skullcap to help reduce stress, and anxiety, and promote a sense of tranquility.

Ingredients:

- 2 tablespoons dried lemon balm leaves
- 1 tablespoon dried passionflower
- 1 tablespoon dried chamomile flowers
- 1 tablespoon dried skullcap
- 1 cup vodka

Method:

1. Combine all the dried herbs in a glass jar.
2. Pour vodka over the herbs, ensuring they are fully covered.
3. Seal the jar tightly and shake well.
4. Store in a cool, dark place for 6-8 weeks, shaking daily.
5. Strain the tincture into a clean bottle.
6. Take 1 teaspoon as needed to promote relaxation and calmness.

Digestive Support Tincture

Description: This digestive support tincture combines peppermint, fennel, ginger, and dandelion to promote healthy digestion, relieve bloating, and ease indigestion.

Ingredients:

- 2 tablespoons dried peppermint leaves
- 1 tablespoon dried fennel seeds
- 1 tablespoon dried dandelion root
- 1 tablespoon dried ginger root
- 1 cup vodka

Method:

1. Combine all the dried herbs in a glass jar.
2. Pour vodka over the herbs, ensuring they are fully covered.
3. Seal the jar tightly and shake well.
4. Store in a cool, dark place for 4-6 weeks, shaking daily.
5. Strain the tincture into a clean bottle.
6. Take 1 teaspoon before or after meals to support digestion.

Respiratory Relief Tincture

Description: This respiratory relief tincture combines mullein, marshmallow root, elecampane root, and thyme to soothe coughs, ease congestion, and support overall respiratory function.

Ingredients:

- 2 tablespoons dried mullein leaves
- 1 tablespoon dried marshmallow root
- 1 tablespoon dried thyme
- 1 tablespoon dried elecampane root
- 1 cup vodka

Method:

1. Combine all the dried herbs in a glass jar.
2. Pour vodka over the herbs, ensuring they are fully covered.
3. Seal the jar tightly and shake well.
4. Store in a cool, dark cupboard for 4-6 weeks, shaking once daily.
5. Strain the tincture into a clean bottle.
6. Take 1-2 teaspoons as needed to support respiratory health and relieve congestion.

Women's Balance Tincture

Description: This women's balance tincture combines vitex berries, dong quai root, black cohosh root, and red raspberry leaves to support hormonal balance and ease menstrual discomfort.

Ingredients:

- 2 tablespoons dried vitex berries
- 1 tablespoon dried dong quai root
- 1 tablespoon dried red raspberry leaves
- 1 tablespoon dried black cohosh root
- 1 cup vodka

Method:

1. Combine all the dried herbs in a glass jar.
2. Pour vodka over the herbs, ensuring they are fully covered.
3. Seal the jar tightly and shake well.
4. Store in a cool, dark cupboard for 6-8 weeks, shaking once daily.
5. Strain the tincture into a clean bottle.
6. Take 1 teaspoon daily to support hormonal balance in women.

Stress Relief Tincture

Description: This tincture combines lemon balm leaves, holy basil leaves, ashwagandha root, and passionflower to help reduce stress and promote relaxation. It can be used as a natural remedy to calm the mind and support overall well-being.

Ingredients:

- 2 tablespoons dried leaves of lemon balm
- 1 tablespoon dried ashwagandha root
- 1 tablespoon dried holy basil leaves
- 1 tablespoon dried passionflower
- 1 cup vodka

Method:

1. Combine all the dried herbs in a glass jar.
2. Pour vodka over the herbs, ensuring they are fully covered.
3. Seal the jar tightly and shake well.
4. Store in a cool, dark cupboard for 4-6 weeks, shaking once daily.
5. Strain the tincture into a clean bottle.
6. Take 1-2 teaspoons as needed to relieve stress and promote relaxation.

Allergy Relief Tincture

Description: This tincture contains nettle leaves, eyebright herb, plantain leaves, and elderflowers, which work synergistically to alleviate allergy symptoms such as sneezing, itching, and congestion. It helps to support a healthy immune response and relieve discomfort caused by seasonal allergies.

Ingredients:

- 1 tablespoon dried eyebright herb
- 2 tablespoons dried nettle leaves
- 1 tablespoon dried plantain leaves
- 1 tablespoon dried elderflowers
- 1 cup vodka

Method:

1. Combine all the dried herbs in a glass jar.
2. Pour vodka over the herbs, ensuring they are fully covered.
3. Seal the jar tightly and shake well.
4. Store in a cool, dark place for 4-6 weeks, shaking daily.
5. Strain the tincture into a clean bottle.
6. Take 1-2 teaspoons as needed to relieve allergy symptoms.

Energy Boost Tincture

Description: This tincture combines ginseng root, maca root, Rhodiola root, and schizandra berries to provide a natural energy boost. It helps combat fatigue, improve stamina, and enhance mental focus, making it ideal for those needing an extra energy lift.

Ingredients:

- 1 tablespoon dried maca root
- 2 tablespoons dried ginseng root
- 1 tablespoon dried Schisandra berries
- 1 tablespoon dried Rhodiola root
- 1 cup vodka

Method:

1. Combine all the dried herbs in a glass jar.
2. Pour vodka over the herbs, ensuring they are fully covered.
3. Seal the jar tightly and shake well.
4. Store in a cool, dark cupboard for 4-6 weeks, shaking once daily.
5. Strain the tincture into a clean bottle.
6. Take 1-2 teaspoons as needed for an energy boost.

Joint Support Tincture

Description: This tincture contains turmeric root, ginger root, Boswellia resin, and devil's claw root, which are well known for their beneficial anti-inflammatory properties. It supports joint health, reduces inflammation, and eases discomfort associated with arthritis or joint-related conditions.

Ingredients:

- 1 tablespoon dried ginger root
- 2 tablespoons dried turmeric root
- 1 tablespoon dried devil's claw root
- 1 tablespoon dried Boswellia resin
- 1 cup vodka

Method:

1. Combine all the dried herbs in a glass jar.
2. Pour vodka over the herbs, ensuring they are fully covered.
3. Seal the jar tightly and shake well.
4. Store in a cool, dark place

Digestive Calming Tincture

Description: This tincture contains peppermint leaves, chamomile flowers, fennel seeds, and lemon balm leaves, which work together to calm digestion and relieve gastrointestinal discomfort. It can be taken after meals to promote digestive health.

Ingredients:

- 1 tablespoon dried chamomile flowers
- 2 tablespoons dried peppermint leaves
- 1 tablespoon dried lemon balm leaves
- 1 tablespoon dried fennel seeds
- 1 cup vodka

Method:

1. Combine all the dried herbs in a glass jar.
2. Pour vodka over the herbs, ensuring they are fully covered.
3. Seal the jar tightly and shake well.
4. Store in a cool, dark cupboard for 4-6 weeks, shaking once daily.
5. Strain the tincture into a clean bottle.
6. Take 1 teaspoon after meals to promote digestive calm.

Immune Boosting Tonic

Description: This tincture combines echinacea root, elderberries, astragalus root, and rose hips to support a healthy immune system. It helps strengthen the body's defenses and prevent illness.

Ingredients:

- 1 tablespoon dried elderberries
- 2 tablespoons dried echinacea root
- 1 tablespoon dried rose hips
- 1 tablespoon dried astragalus root
- 1 cup vodka

Method:

1. Combine all the dried herbs in a glass jar.
2. Pour vodka over the herbs, ensuring they are fully covered.
3. Seal the jar tightly and shake well.
4. Store in a cool, dark cupboard for 4-6 weeks, shaking once daily.
5. Strain the tincture into a clean bottle.
6. Take 1-2 teaspoons daily to support immune function.

Anxiety Relief Tincture

Description: This tincture contains lemon balm leaves, chamomile flowers, skullcap, and lavender flowers, which have calming properties to help reduce anxiety and promote relaxation. It can be used during times of stress or nervousness.

Ingredients:

- 2 tablespoons dried lemon balm leaves
- 1 tablespoon dried lavender flowers
- 1 tablespoon dried chamomile flowers
- 1 tablespoon dried skullcap
- 1 cup vodka

Method:

1. Combine all the dried herbs in a glass jar.
2. Pour vodka over the herbs, ensuring they are fully covered.
3. Seal the jar tightly and shake well.
4. Store in a cool, dark cupboard for 6-8 weeks, shaking once daily.
5. Strain the tincture into a clean bottle.
6. Take 1-2 teaspoons as needed to reduce anxiety.

Sleep Support Tincture

Description: This tincture combines valerian root, passionflower, chamomile flowers, and lemon balm leaves to promote restful sleep. It can be taken before bedtime to support relaxation and enhance sleep quality.

Ingredients:

- 1 tablespoon dried chamomile flowers
- 2 tablespoons dried valerian root
- 1 tablespoon dried passionflower
- 1 tablespoon dried lemon balm leaves
- 1 cup vodka

Method:

1. Combine all the dried herbs in a glass jar.
2. Pour vodka over the herbs, ensuring they are fully covered.
3. Seal the jar tightly and shake well.
4. Store in a cool, dark cupboard for 4-6 weeks, shaking once daily.
5. Strain the tincture into a clean bottle.
6. Take 1-2 teaspoons before bedtime to promote restful sleep.

Hormonal Balance Tincture (for Women)

Description: This tincture contains black cohosh root, dong quai root, vitex berries, and red clover blossoms, which help support hormonal balance in women. It can be used to alleviate symptoms associated with menstrual irregularities and menopause.

Ingredients:

- 1 tablespoon dried dong quai root
- 2 tablespoons dried black cohosh root
- 1 tablespoon dried red clover blossoms
- 1 tablespoon dried vitex berries
- 1 cup vodka

Method:

1. Combine all the dried herbs in a glass jar.
2. Pour vodka over the herbs, ensuring they are fully covered.
3. Seal the jar tightly and shake well.
4. Store in a cool, dark cupboard for 4-6 weeks, shaking once daily.
5. Strain the tincture into a clean bottle.
6. Take 1-2 teaspoons daily to support hormonal balance.

Focus and Clarity Tincture

Description: This tincture combines gotu kola leaves, ginkgo biloba leaves, rosemary leaves, and lemon verbena leaves, which are known for their cognitive-enhancing properties. It helps improve focus, concentration, and mental clarity, making it beneficial for students or those needing mental sharpness.

Ingredients:

- 2 tablespoons dried gotu kola leaves
- 1 tablespoon dried lemon verbena leaves
- 1 tablespoon dried ginkgo biloba leaves
- 1 tablespoon dried rosemary leaves
- 1 cup vodka

Method:

1. Combine all the dried herbs in a glass jar.
2. Pour vodka over the herbs, ensuring they are fully covered.
3. Seal the jar tightly and shake well.
4. Store in a cool, dark cupboard for 4-6 weeks, shaking it daily.
5. Strain the tincture into a clean bottle.
6. Take 1-2 teaspoons as needed to improve focus and mental clarity.

Calming Nervous System Tincture

Description: This tincture contains oats, passionflower, skullcap, and lemon balm leaves, which have calming and soothing properties to support the nervous system. It can be used during times of stress, anxiety, or restlessness.

Ingredients:

- 2 tablespoons dried oats
- 1 tablespoon dried lemon balm leaves
- 1 tablespoon dried passionflower
- 1 tablespoon dried skullcap
- 1 cup vodka

Method:

1. Combine all the dried herbs in a glass jar.
2. Pour vodka over the herbs, ensuring they are fully covered.
3. Seal the jar tightly and shake well.
4. Store in a cool, dark cupboard for 6-8 weeks, shaking it daily.
5. Strain the tincture into a clean bottle.
6. Take 1-2 teaspoons as needed to calm and soothe the nervous system.

Respiratory Support Tincture

Description: This tincture combines mullein leaves, elecampane root, thyme leaves, and marshmallow root to support respiratory health. It helps soothe coughs, promote clear breathing, and alleviates congestion.

Ingredients:

- 2 tablespoons dried mullein leaves
- 1 tablespoon dried marshmallow root
- 1 tablespoon dried elecampane root
- 1 tablespoon dried thyme leaves
- 1 cup vodka

Method:

1. Combine all the dried herbs in a glass jar.
2. Pour vodka over the herbs, ensuring they are fully covered.
3. Seal the jar tightly and shake well.
4. Store in a cool, dark cupboard for 4-6 weeks, shaking it daily.
5. Strain the tincture into a clean bottle.
6. Take 1-2 teaspoons as needed to support respiratory health.

Mood Balancing Tincture

Description: This tincture contains St. John's wort, lavender flowers, lemon balm leaves, and passionflower, which work synergistically to support emotional well-being and balance mood. It can be used during periods of mild depression or mood fluctuations.

Ingredients:

- 2 tablespoons dried St. John's wort
- 1 tablespoon dried lemon balm leaves
- 1 tablespoon dried passionflower
- 1 tablespoon dried lavender flowers
- 1 cup vodka

Method:

1. Combine all the dried herbs in a glass jar.
2. Pour vodka over the herbs, ensuring they are fully covered.
3. Seal the jar tightly and shake well.
4. Store in a cool, dark cupboard for 4-6 weeks, shaking once daily.
5. Strain the tincture into a clean bottle.
6. Take 1-2 teaspoons daily to promote mood balance.

Hair and Scalp Nourishing Tincture

Description: This tincture combines horsetail herb, nettle leaves, rosemary leaves, and lavender flowers, which are beneficial for maintaining healthy hair and scalp. It can be used topically as a scalp rinse or added to hair care products.

Ingredients:

- 2 tablespoons dried horsetail herb
- 1 tablespoon dried nettle leaves
- 1 tablespoon dried rosemary leaves
- 1 tablespoon dried lavender flowers
- 1 cup vodka

Method:

1. Combine all the dried herbs in a glass jar.
2. Pour vodka over the herbs, ensuring they are fully covered.
3. Seal the jar tightly and shake well.
4. Store in a cool, dark place for 4-6 weeks, shaking daily.
5. Strain the tincture into a clean bottle.
6. Dilute with water and use as a scalp rinse or add a few drops to hair care products.

Circulation Support Tincture

Description: This tincture contains hawthorn berries, ginger root, cayenne pepper, and ginkgo biloba leaves, which support healthy circulation and cardiovascular function. It can be used to improve blood flow and promote overall cardiovascular health.

Ingredients:

- 2 tablespoons dried hawthorn berries
- 1 tablespoon dried ginkgo biloba leaves
- 1 tablespoon dried ginger root
- 1 teaspoon dried cayenne pepper
- 1 cup vodka

Method:

1. Combine all the dried herbs in a glass jar.
2. Pour vodka over the herbs, ensuring they are fully covered.
3. Seal the jar tightly and shake well.
4. Store in a cool, dark cupboard for 4-6 weeks, shaking once daily.
5. Strain the tincture into a clean bottle.
6. Take 1-2 teaspoons daily to support healthy circulation and cardiovascular function.

Detox Support Tincture

Description: This tincture combines dandelion root, burdock root, milk thistle seeds, and yellow dock root to support the body's natural detoxification processes. It helps cleanse the liver and promote overall detoxification.

Ingredients:

- 2 tablespoons dried dandelion root
- 1 tablespoon dried yellow dock root
- 1 tablespoon dried burdock root
- 1 tablespoon dried milk thistle seeds
- 1 cup vodka

Method:

1. Combine all the dried herbs in a glass jar.
2. Pour vodka over the herbs, ensuring they are fully covered.
3. Seal the jar tightly and shake well.
4. Store in a cool, dark cupboard for 4-6 weeks, shaking it once daily.
5. Strain the tincture into a clean bottle.
6. Take 1-2 teaspoons daily to support detoxification.

Memory and Cognitive Function Tincture

Description: This tincture contains gotu kola leaves, ginkgo biloba leaves, rosemary leaves, and lemon balm leaves, which are known to enhance memory and cognitive function. It can be used to support mental clarity and focus.

Ingredients:

- 2 tablespoons dried gotu kola leaves
- 1 tablespoon dried lemon balm leaves
- 1 tablespoon dried ginkgo biloba leaves
- 1 tablespoon dried rosemary leaves
- 1 cup vodka

Method:

1. Combine all the dried herbs in a glass jar.
2. Pour vodka over the herbs, ensuring they are fully covered.
3. Seal the jar tightly and shake well.
4. Store in a cool, dark cupboard for 4-6 weeks, shaking it once daily.
5. Strain the tincture into a clean bottle.
6. Take 1-2 teaspoons as needed to support memory and cognitive function.

Calming Sleep Tincture

Description: This tincture combines valerian root, passionflower, chamomile flowers, and lavender flowers to promote deep, restful sleep. It can be used to ease insomnia and improve sleep quality.

Ingredients:

- 2 tablespoons dried valerian root
- 1 tablespoon dried lavender flowers
- 1 tablespoon dried passionflower
- 1 tablespoon dried chamomile flowers
- 1 cup vodka

Method:

1. Combine all the dried herbs in a glass jar.
2. Pour vodka over the herbs, ensuring they are fully covered.
3. Seal the jar tightly and shake well.
4. Store in a cool, dark cupboard for 4-6 weeks, shaking it once daily.
5. Strain the tincture into a clean bottle.
6. Take 1-2 teaspoons before bedtime to promote calming sleep.

Skin Healing Tincture

Description: This tincture contains calendula flowers, plantain leaves, comfrey root, and chamomile flowers, which have soothing and healing properties for the skin. It can be applied topically to promote wound healing and relieve skin irritations.

Ingredients:

- 2 tablespoons dried calendula flowers
- 1 tablespoon dried chamomile flowers
- 1 tablespoon dried plantain leaves
- 1 tablespoon dried comfrey root
- 1 cup vodka

Method:

1. Combine all the dried herbs in a glass jar.
2. Pour vodka over the herbs, ensuring they are fully covered.
3. Seal the jar tightly and shake well.
4. Store in a cool, dark cupboard for 4-6 weeks, shaking it once daily.
5. Strain the tincture into a clean bottle.
6. Apply topically to affected areas for skin healing and relief.

Joint Support Tincture

Description: This tincture combines turmeric root, ginger root, Boswellia resin, and devil's claw root, which have anti-inflammatory properties and can help support joint health. It may be beneficial for individuals experiencing joint pain or stiffness.

Ingredients:

- 2 tablespoons dried turmeric root
- 1 tablespoon dried devil's claw root
- 1 tablespoon dried ginger root
- 1 tablespoon dried Boswellia resin
- 1 cup vodka

Method:

1. Combine all the dried herbs in a glass jar.
2. Pour vodka over the herbs, ensuring they are fully covered.
3. Seal the jar tightly and shake well.
4. Store in a cool, dark cupboard for 4-6 weeks, shaking it once daily.
5. Strain the tincture into a clean bottle.
6. Take 1-2 teaspoons daily to support joint health.

Eye Health Tincture

Description: This tincture contains bilberry fruit, eyebright herb, ginkgo biloba leaves, and chamomile flowers, which are known for their beneficial effects on eye health. It can be used to support healthy vision and relieve eye strain.

Ingredients:

- 2 tablespoons dried bilberry fruit
- 1 tablespoon dried chamomile flowers
- 1 tablespoon dried eyebright herb
- 1 tablespoon dried ginkgo biloba leaves
- 1 cup vodka

Method:

1. Combine all the dried herbs in a glass jar.
2. Pour vodka over the herbs, ensuring they are fully covered.
3. Seal the jar tightly and shake well.
4. Store in a cool, dark cupboard for 4-6 weeks, shaking it once daily.
5. Strain the tincture into a clean bottle.
6. Take 1-2 teaspoons daily to support eye health.

Digestive Bitters Tincture

Description: This tincture combines dandelion root, gentian root, fennel seeds, and orange peel, which are traditional digestive bitters. It can be used to support healthy digestion and stimulate digestive enzymes.

Ingredients:

- 2 tablespoons dried dandelion root
- 1 tablespoon dried orange peel
- 1 tablespoon dried gentian root
- 1 tablespoon dried fennel seeds
- 1 cup vodka

Method:

1. Combine all the dried herbs in a glass jar.
2. Pour vodka over the herbs, ensuring they are fully covered.
3. Seal the jar tightly and shake well.
4. Store in a cool, dark cupboard for 4-6 weeks, shaking it once daily.
5. Strain the tincture into a clean bottle.
6. Take 1 teaspoon before meals to support healthy digestion.

Immune Boosting Tincture

Description: This tincture contains echinacea root, elderberry fruit, astragalus root, and reishi mushroom, which are known for their immune-boosting properties. It can be used to support a healthy immune system and prevent seasonal illnesses.

Ingredients:

- 2 tablespoons dried echinacea root
- 1 tablespoon dried reishi mushroom
- 1 tablespoon dried elderberry fruit
- 1 tablespoon dried astragalus root
- 1 tablespoon dried reishi mushroom
- 1 cup vodka

Method:

1. Combine all the dried herbs in a glass jar.
2. Pour vodka over the herbs, ensuring they are fully covered.
3. Seal the jar tightly and shake well.
4. Store in a cool, dark cupboard for 4-6 weeks, shaking it once daily.
5. Strain the tincture into a clean bottle.
6. Take 1-2 teaspoons daily to support immune health.

Respiratory Support Tincture

Description: This tincture combines mullein leaves, elecampane root, marshmallow root, and licorice root, which have soothing and expectorant properties for the respiratory system. It can be used to support respiratory health and relieve coughs.

Ingredients:

- 2 tablespoons dried mullein leaves
- 1 tablespoon dried licorice root
- 1 tablespoon dried elecampane root
- 1 tablespoon dried marshmallow root
- 1 cup vodka

Method:

1. Combine all the dried herbs in a glass jar.
2. Pour vodka over the herbs, ensuring they are fully covered.
3. Seal the jar tightly and shake well.
4. Store in a cool, dark cupboard for 4-6 weeks, shaking it daily.
5. Strain the tincture into a clean bottle.
6. Take 1-2 teaspoons as needed to support respiratory health.

IMPORTANT! Remember to consult with a healthcare professional before using these herbal tinctures, especially if you have any underlying health conditions or are taking medications already. There is a potential that natural supplements can interact with any drugs you are already taking.

Blood Sugar Balancing Tincture

Description: This tincture combines cinnamon bark, Gymnema sylvestre leaves, fenugreek seeds, and bitter melon to support healthy blood sugar levels. It may assist in balancing glucose metabolism and promoting insulin sensitivity.

Ingredients:

- 2 tablespoons dried cinnamon bark
- 1 tablespoon dried bitter melon
- 1 tablespoon dried Gymnema sylvestre leaves
- 1 tablespoon dried fenugreek seeds
- 1 cup vodka

Method:

1. Combine all the dried herbs in a glass jar.
2. Pour vodka over the herbs, ensuring they are fully covered.
3. Seal the jar tightly and shake well.
4. Store in a cool, dark cupboard for 4-6 weeks, shaking it daily.
5. Strain the tincture into a clean bottle.
6. Take 1-2 teaspoons daily to support blood sugar balance.

Pancreatic Support Tincture

Description: This tincture contains blueberry leaves, bilberry leaves, goat's rue, and turmeric root, which are known for their potential to support pancreatic health and insulin production. It can be used to complement a healthy lifestyle for blood sugar management.

Ingredients:

- 2 tablespoons dried blueberry leaves
- 1 tablespoon dried turmeric root
- 1 tablespoon dried bilberry leaves
- 1 tablespoon dried goat's rue
- 1 cup vodka

Method:

1. Combine all the dried herbs in a glass jar.
2. Pour vodka over the herbs, ensuring they are fully covered.
3. Seal the jar tightly and shake well.
4. Store in a cool, dark cupboard for 4-6 weeks, shaking it once daily.
5. Strain the tincture into a clean bottle.
6. Take 1-2 teaspoons daily to support pancreatic health and blood sugar regulation.

IMPORTANT! As always, it's important to consult with a healthcare professional before incorporating herbal remedies into your routine, especially if you have any underlying health conditions or are taking medications related to blood sugar management.

Ashwagandha and Lavender Stress Relief Tincture

Description: This tincture combines lemon balm leaves, ashwagandha root, passionflower, and lavender flowers, which are known for their calming and stress-relieving properties. It can be used to promote relaxation and ease symptoms of stress and anxiety.

Ingredients:

- 2 tablespoons dried lemon balm leaves
- 1 tablespoon dried lavender flowers
- 1 tablespoon dried ashwagandha root
- 1 tablespoon dried passionflower
- 1 tablespoon dried lavender flowers
- 1 cup vodka

Method:

1. Combine all the dried herbs in a glass jar.
2. Pour vodka over the herbs, ensuring they are fully covered.
3. Seal the jar tightly and shake well.
4. Store in a cool, dark cupboard for 4-6 weeks, shaking once daily.
5. Strain the tincture into a clean bottle.
6. Take 1-2 teaspoons as needed to support stress relief and relaxation.

Dong Quai and Mace Hormonal Balance Tincture (woman)

Description: This tincture contains vitex berries (chasteberry), dong quai root, black cohosh root, and maca root, which are traditionally used to support hormonal balance in women. It may be beneficial for managing symptoms associated with hormonal fluctuations.

Ingredients:

- 2 tablespoons dried vitex berries (chasteberry)
- 1 tablespoon dried maca root
- 1 tablespoon dried dong quai root
- 1 tablespoon dried black cohosh root
- 1 cup vodka

Method:

1. Combine all the dried herbs in a glass jar.
2. Pour vodka over the herbs, ensuring they are fully covered.
3. Seal the jar tightly and shake well.
4. Store in a cool, dark cupboard for 4-6 weeks, shaking it once daily.
5. Strain the tincture into a clean bottle.
6. Take 1-2 teaspoons daily to support hormonal balance.

Peppermint Ginger Digestive Support Tincture

Description: This tincture combines peppermint leaves, ginger root, fennel seeds, and chamomile flowers, which have soothing and carminative properties for the digestive system. It can be used to alleviate digestive discomfort and promote healthy digestion.

Ingredients:

- 2 tablespoons dried peppermint leaves
- 1 tablespoon dried chamomile flowers
- 1 tablespoon dried ginger root
- 1 tablespoon dried fennel seeds
- 1 cup vodka

Method:

1. Combine all the dried herbs in a glass jar.
2. Pour vodka over the herbs, ensuring they are fully covered.
3. Seal the jar tightly and shake well.
4. Store in a cool, dark cupboard for 4-6 weeks, shaking it once daily.
5. Strain the tincture into a clean bottle.
6. Take 1 teaspoon before or after meals to support healthy digestion.

Energy Boost Tincture 2

Description: This tincture contains ginseng root, Rhodiola root, maca root, and licorice root, which are known for their potential to increase energy and combat fatigue. It can be used to promote mental and physical vitality.

Ingredients:

- 2 tablespoons dried ginseng root
- 1 tablespoon dried licorice root
- 1 tablespoon dried rhodiola root
- 1 tablespoon dried maca root
- 1 cup vodka

Method:

1. Combine all the dried herbs in a glass jar.
2. Pour vodka over the herbs, ensuring they are fully covered.
3. Seal the jar tightly and shake well.
4. Store in a cool, dark cupboard for 4-6 weeks, shaking it daily.
5. Strain the tincture into a clean bottle.
6. Take 1-2 teaspoons daily to support energy and vitality.

Brain Health Tincture 2

Description: This tincture combines gotu kola leaves, rosemary leaves, ginkgo biloba leaves, and holy basil leaves, which are known for their potential cognitive-enhancing properties. It can be used to support brain health and memory function.

Ingredients:

- 2 tablespoons dried gotu kola leaves
- 1 tablespoon dried holy basil leaves
- 1 tablespoon dried rosemary leaves
- 1 tablespoon dried ginkgo biloba leaves
- 1 cup vodka

Method:

1. Combine all the dried herbs in a glass jar.
2. Pour vodka over the herbs, ensuring they are fully covered.
3. Seal the jar tightly and shake well.
4. Store in a cool, dark cupboard for 4-6 weeks, shaking it once daily.
5. Strain the tincture into a clean bottle.
6. Take 1-2 teaspoons daily to support brain health and cognitive function.

Remember to consult with a healthcare professional before using these herbal tinctures, especially if you have any underlying health conditions or are taking medications.

I HOPE YOU HAVE ENJOYED the recipes and this book or ebook! If you enjoyed it, could you please leave a review on the online retailer site or app where you got your copy at? Thanks so much – I really appreciate it!

Don't miss out!

Visit the website below and you can sign up to receive emails whenever Kathy Wyatt publishes a new book. There's no charge and no obligation.

https://books2read.com/r/B-A-FLDG-HLILC

BOOKS 2 READ

Connecting independent readers to independent writers.

Also by Kathy Wyatt

Homesteading Freedom

Beginner's Guide to Essential Oils and Herbal Tinctures: DIY Natural Remedies with Herbs, Aromatherapy Recipes, Infused Oils, and Much More!

A Relaxing Country Christmas Cookbook: Holiday Recipes you Should Have got From Your Grandmother!

Standalone

Herbal Tinctures for Beginners: Natural Remedies for Healing Recipes and More